Diet For Acid Reflux Disorder

Surprising Foods to Say Goodbye to Acid Reflux and GERD forever

Maya   Arlo

TABLE OF CONTENTS

Chapter 1: Introduction to Acid Reflux Disorder and GERD

Chapter 2: The Link between Diet and Acid Reflux: How the foods we eat affect our digestive system

Chapter 3: Acid Reflux Triggers: Common foods and drinks that trigger symptoms

Chapter 4: Acid Reflux-Friendly Foods: The best foods to eat to prevent acid reflux and reduce symptoms

Chapter 5: Meal Planning for Acid Reflux: How to plan healthy meals that are easy on the digestive system

Chapter 6: Lifestyle Changes for Managing Acid Reflux: Tips for managing stress, exercising, and sleeping to reduce symptoms

Chapter 7: Recipes for a Reflux-Friendly Diet: Delicious and Nutritious Meal Ideas for Breakfast, Lunch, Dinner, and Snacks that are Gentle on the Digestive System

Chapter 1

Introduction to Acid Reflux Disorder and GERD

Acid reflux disorder, also known as gastroesophageal reflux disease (GERD), is a common condition that affects millions of people worldwide. The condition occurs when the stomach acid flows back up into the esophagus, causing discomfort, pain, and irritation.

In this chapter, we will discuss the symptoms and causes of acid reflux disorder, as well as the various treatment options available.

Symptoms of Acid Reflux Disorder

The most common symptom of acid reflux disorder is heartburn, which is characterized by a burning sensation in the chest that may radiate to the throat and neck. Other symptoms of the condition include regurgitation, nausea, difficulty swallowing, and a persistent cough.

Symptoms of acid reflux disorder may be worse at night or when lying down, as gravity is no longer able to keep the stomach acid in the stomach. Some individuals may also experience symptoms after consuming certain foods or drinks, such as spicy foods, caffeine, and alcohol.

Causes of Acid Reflux Disorder

Acid reflux disorder occurs when the lower esophageal sphincter (LES), a muscle that separates the stomach from the esophagus, fails to close properly. When the LES is weak or relaxed, the stomach acid can flow back up into the esophagus, causing irritation and inflammation.

Several factors can contribute to the development of acid reflux disorder, including obesity, smoking, and pregnancy. Certain medications, such as aspirin and ibuprofen, can also weaken the LES and increase the risk of developing the condition.

Treatment Options for Acid Reflux Disorder

There are several treatment options available for acid reflux disorder, including lifestyle changes, medications, and surgery.

Lifestyle Changes: Making certain lifestyle changes can help reduce the symptoms of acid reflux disorder. These changes include avoiding trigger foods and drinks, losing weight, and quitting smoking. Elevating the head of the bed and avoiding eating before bedtime can also help reduce symptoms.

Medications: Several medications can help relieve the symptoms of acid reflux disorder, including antacids, H2 blockers, and proton pump inhibitors (PPIs). Antacids work by neutralizing stomach acid, while H2 blockers and PPIs reduce the amount of acid produced by the stomach.

Surgery: In severe cases of acid reflux disorder, surgery may be necessary to strengthen the LES and prevent the stomach acid from flowing back up into the esophagus. The most common type of surgery for acid reflux disorder is a fundoplication, in which the upper part of the stomach is wrapped around the LES to strengthen the muscle.

Acid reflux disorder is a common condition that can cause discomfort and pain. Understanding the symptoms and causes of the condition is essential for effective treatment. Lifestyle changes, medications, and surgery are all treatment options that can help relieve the symptoms of acid reflux disorder and improve quality of life. It is important to consult with a healthcare professional to determine the best course of treatment for individual cases of acid reflux disorder.

Chapter

2

The Link between Diet and Acid Reflux: How the foods we eat affect our digestive system

Diet plays a significant role in the development and management of acid reflux disorder. Certain foods and drinks can trigger symptoms, while others can help prevent or reduce them. In this chapter, we will discuss the link between diet and acid reflux and how the foods we eat affect our digestive system.

Foods and Drinks that Trigger Acid Reflux

Several foods and drinks can trigger the symptoms of acid reflux disorder by relaxing the LES or increasing the production of stomach acid. Some common trigger foods and drinks include:

Spicy foods: Spicy foods can irritate the lining of the esophagus and cause discomfort and pain.

Citrus fruits and juices: Citrus fruits and juices are highly acidic and can increase the production of stomach acid, leading to symptoms of acid reflux.

Tomatoes and tomato-based products: Tomatoes and tomato-based products, such as pasta sauce and ketchup, are highly acidic and can trigger symptoms of acid reflux.

Carbonated beverages: Carbonated beverages can increase the pressure on the LES, causing it to relax and allowing stomach acid to flow back up into the esophagus.

Alcohol: Alcohol can irritate the lining of the esophagus and increase the production of stomach acid, leading to symptoms of acid reflux.

Foods and Drinks that Help Prevent Acid Reflux

On the other hand, there are several foods and drinks that can help prevent or reduce the symptoms of acid reflux disorder. These foods and drinks include:

Low-fat dairy products: Low-fat dairy products, such as milk and yogurt, can help reduce the production of stomach acid and prevent symptoms of acid reflux.

Lean protein: Lean protein sources, such as chicken and fish, are less likely to trigger symptoms of acid reflux than high-fat meats.

Non-citrus fruits: Non-citrus fruits, such as bananas and apples, are low in acid and can help reduce symptoms of acid reflux.

Vegetables: Vegetables, especially leafy greens, are low in acid and can help reduce the production of stomach acid.

Water: Drinking plenty of water can help dilute stomach acid and prevent symptoms of acid reflux.

The Digestive System and Acid Reflux

Understanding the digestive system can help individuals with acid reflux disorder make better dietary choices. The digestive system begins with the mouth and ends with the anus, and includes several organs and glands that work together to break down food and absorb nutrients.

The stomach is a muscular sac that mixes food with stomach acid and digestive enzymes to break it down into a liquid-like substance called chyme. The LES separates the stomach from the esophagus and opens to allow food to enter the stomach, then closes to prevent the stomach acid from flowing back up into the esophagus.

When the LES is weak or relaxed, the stomach acid can flow back up into the esophagus, causing irritation and inflammation. By making dietary choices that reduce the production of stomach acid and prevent the LES from relaxing, individuals with acid reflux disorder can reduce the symptoms of the condition.

Diet plays a significant role in the development and management of acid reflux disorder. Certain foods and drinks can trigger symptoms, while others can help prevent or reduce them. By understanding the link between diet and acid reflux and how the foods we eat affect our digestive system, individuals with acid reflux disorder can make better dietary choices to reduce the symptoms of the condition. It is important to consult with a healthcare professional to determine a personalized diet plan that works best for individual cases of acid reflux disorder.

Chapter

3

Acid Reflux Triggers: Common foods and drinks that trigger symptoms

Acid reflux disorder is a condition that occurs when the lower esophageal sphincter (LES) fails to close properly, allowing stomach acid to flow back up into the esophagus. Certain foods and drinks can trigger the symptoms of acid reflux, making it important for individuals with the condition to be aware of their triggers. In this chapter, we will discuss the common foods and drinks that can trigger symptoms of acid reflux.

High-fat Foods

High-fat foods, such as fried foods, fatty meats, and buttery or creamy dishes, can cause the LES to relax, allowing stomach acid to flow back up into the esophagus. These foods take longer to digest, which can also increase the production of stomach acid and lead to symptoms of acid reflux.

Citrus Fruits

Citrus fruits, such as oranges, grapefruits, and lemons, are highly acidic and can increase the production of stomach acid, making them a common trigger for acid reflux symptoms. Citrus juices, such as orange juice and grapefruit juice, can also trigger symptoms.

Tomatoes

Tomatoes and tomato-based products, such as pasta sauce and ketchup, are highly acidic and can trigger symptoms of acid reflux. Cooking tomatoes can reduce their acidity, making them less likely to trigger symptoms.

Spicy Foods

Spicy foods, such as hot peppers, chili, and curry, can irritate the lining of the esophagus and cause discomfort and pain. Spicy foods can also increase the production of stomach acid, making them a common trigger for acid reflux symptoms.

Carbonated Beverages

Carbonated beverages, such as soda and sparkling water, can increase the pressure on the LES, causing it to relax and allowing stomach acid to flow back up into the esophagus. This can lead to symptoms of acid reflux, such as heartburn and regurgitation.

Alcohol

Alcohol can irritate the lining of the esophagus and increase the production of stomach acid, leading to symptoms of acid reflux. Beer, wine, and hard liquor can all trigger symptoms, but individuals may find that certain types of alcohol are worse than others.

Caffeine

Caffeine can increase the production of stomach acid and relax the LES, making it a common trigger for acid reflux symptoms. Coffee, tea, and soda all contain caffeine and can trigger symptoms.

Chocolate

Chocolate contains both caffeine and a compound called theobromine, which can relax the LES and cause symptoms of acid reflux. Dark chocolate is higher in theobromine than milk chocolate, making it more likely to trigger symptoms.

Peppermint

Peppermint can relax the LES and cause symptoms of acid reflux. This includes peppermint tea and peppermint oil, which are often used to soothe digestive issues but can actually worsen acid reflux symptoms.

Onions and Garlic

Onions and garlic can increase the production of stomach acid and relax the LES, making them common triggers for acid reflux symptoms. Cooking onions and garlic can reduce their acidity and make them less likely to trigger symptoms.

Certain foods and drinks can trigger the symptoms of acid reflux, making it important for individuals with the condition to be aware of their triggers. High-fat foods, citrus fruits, tomatoes, spicy foods, carbonated beverages, alcohol, caffeine, chocolate, peppermint, and onions and garlic are all common triggers for acid reflux symptoms. By identifying and avoiding trigger foods, individuals with acid reflux disorder can reduce the frequency and severity of their symptoms. It is important to consult with a healthcare professional to determine a personalized diet plan that works best for individual cases of acid reflux disorder.

Chapter 4

Acid Reflux-Friendly Foods: The best foods to eat to prevent acid reflux and reduce symptoms

While certain foods can trigger the symptoms of acid reflux, there are also foods that can help prevent and reduce symptoms. In this chapter, we will discuss the best foods to eat to prevent acid reflux and reduce symptoms.

Non-Citrus Fruits

Non-citrus fruits, such as bananas, melons, and apples, are low in acid and can help neutralize stomach acid. They are also high in fiber, which can help regulate digestion and prevent constipation, a common trigger for acid reflux.

Vegetables

Vegetables are high in fiber and low in fat, making them a great choice for individuals with acid reflux disorder. Green vegetables, such as spinach, kale, and broccoli, are particularly beneficial,

as they are low in acid and high in
nutrients.

Lean Proteins

Lean proteins, such as chicken, fish, and
tofu, are easy to digest and can help
regulate digestion. They are also low in
fat, which can help prevent the relaxation
of the LES and the flow of stomach acid
back up into the esophagus.

Whole Grains

Whole grains, such as oatmeal, brown
rice, and whole wheat bread, are high in
fiber and can help regulate digestion.
They are also low in fat, making them a
good choice for individuals with acid
reflux disorder.

Low-Fat Dairy Products

Low-fat dairy products, such as skim milk, yogurt, and cheese, are a good source of calcium and protein, which can help strengthen the LES and prevent the flow of stomach acid back up into the esophagus. However, individuals with acid reflux should avoid high-fat dairy products, such as whole milk and cream.

Ginger

Ginger has natural anti-inflammatory properties and can help soothe the lining of the esophagus. It can be consumed as a tea or added to dishes as a spice.

Aloe Vera

Aloe vera has natural anti-inflammatory properties and can help soothe the lining of the esophagus. Aloe vera juice can be consumed before meals to help prevent symptoms of acid reflux.

Oatmeal

Oatmeal is a great source of fiber and can help regulate digestion. It is also low in fat, making it a good choice for individuals with acid reflux disorder.

Almonds

Almonds are a good source of healthy fats and protein, making them a great snack for individuals with acid reflux disorder. However, individuals with acid reflux should avoid high-fat nuts, such as cashews and peanuts.

Chamomile Tea

Chamomile tea has natural anti-inflammatory properties and can help soothe the lining of the esophagus. It can be consumed before bedtime to help prevent symptoms of acid reflux.

Certain foods can help prevent and reduce the symptoms of acid reflux. Non-citrus fruits, vegetables, lean proteins, whole grains, low-fat dairy products, ginger, aloe vera, oatmeal, almonds, and chamomile tea are all great choices for individuals with acid reflux disorder. By incorporating these acid reflux-friendly foods into their diet, individuals can help regulate digestion and prevent the flow of stomach acid back up into the esophagus. It is important to consult with a healthcare professional to determine a personalized diet plan that works best for individual cases of acid reflux disorder.

Chapter 5

Meal Planning for Acid Reflux: How to plan healthy meals that are easy on the digestive system

Meal planning is an important part of managing acid reflux disorder. By planning meals ahead of time, individuals can ensure that they are consuming a balanced diet that is easy on their digestive system. In this chapter, we will discuss how to plan healthy meals that are easy on the digestive system for individuals with acid reflux disorder.

Start with a Protein

When planning meals, it is important to start with a protein. Lean proteins, such as chicken, fish, and tofu, are easy to digest and can help regulate digestion. They are also low in fat, which can help prevent the relaxation of the LES and the flow of stomach acid back up into the esophagus.

Incorporate Non-Citrus Fruits and Vegetables

Non-citrus fruits, such as bananas, melons, and apples, are low in acid and can help neutralize stomach acid. They are also high in fiber, which can help regulate digestion and prevent constipation, a common trigger for acid reflux. Vegetables, such as spinach, kale, and broccoli, are also high in fiber and low in fat, making them a great choice for individuals with acid reflux disorder.

Choose Whole Grains

Whole grains, such as oatmeal, brown rice, and whole wheat bread, are high in fiber and can help regulate digestion. They are also low in fat, making them a good choice for individuals with acid reflux disorder. When choosing grains, it is important to avoid those that are high in fat, such as croissants and biscuits.

Limit High-Fat Foods

High-fat foods, such as fried foods, cheese, and cream-based sauces, can cause the LES to relax, allowing stomach acid to flow back up into the esophagus. When planning meals, it is important to limit high-fat foods and opt for low-fat alternatives instead.

Use Spices and Herbs for Flavor

When planning meals for acid reflux, it is important to use spices and herbs for flavor instead of high-fat sauces and condiments. Spices such as ginger, cumin, and turmeric can also help regulate digestion and reduce inflammation in the digestive tract.

Opt for Small, Frequent Meals

Eating smaller, more frequent meals throughout the day can help prevent the stomach from becoming too full, which can trigger symptoms of acid reflux. It is important to avoid eating large meals before bedtime, as this can increase the risk of symptoms during the night.

Stay Hydrated

Drinking plenty of water throughout the day can help regulate digestion and prevent constipation, a common trigger for acid reflux. It is important to avoid beverages that can trigger symptoms of acid reflux, such as coffee, alcohol, and carbonated beverages.

Meal planning is an important part of managing acid reflux disorder. By starting with a protein, incorporating non-citrus fruits and vegetables, choosing whole grains, limiting high-fat foods, using spices and herbs for flavor, opting for small, frequent meals, and staying hydrated, individuals can plan healthy meals that are easy on their digestive system. It is important to work with a healthcare professional to develop a personalized diet plan that takes individual triggers and symptoms into account. By following a healthy diet and avoiding triggers, individuals can manage their acid reflux symptoms and improve their overall digestive health.

Chapter 6

Lifestyle Changes for Managing Acid Reflux: Tips for managing stress, exercising, and sleeping to reduce symptoms

In addition to making dietary changes, lifestyle modifications can also play a significant role in managing acid reflux disorder. In this chapter, we will discuss some tips for managing stress, exercising, and sleeping to reduce symptoms of acid reflux.

Manage Stress

Stress can contribute to acid reflux by increasing the production of stomach acid and causing the LES to relax. To manage stress, individuals can try relaxation techniques, such as meditation, deep breathing exercises, and yoga. Engaging in hobbies and spending time with loved ones can also help reduce stress levels.

Exercise Regularly

Regular exercise can help improve digestion and reduce stress levels, both of which can contribute to acid reflux. However, it is important to avoid exercising immediately after meals, as this can increase the risk of symptoms. Instead, individuals should wait at least 2-3 hours after eating before engaging in exercise.

Maintain a Healthy Weight

Excess weight can put pressure on the stomach, causing the LES to relax and allowing stomach acid to flow back up into the esophagus. Maintaining a healthy weight through diet and exercise can help reduce symptoms of acid reflux.

Elevate the Head of the Bed

Elevating the head of the bed by 6-8 inches can help prevent stomach acid from flowing back up into the esophagus while sleeping. This can be achieved by placing blocks under the legs of the bed or by using a wedge-shaped pillow.

Sleep on Your Left Side

Sleeping on the left side can help reduce symptoms of acid reflux by preventing stomach acid from flowing back up into the esophagus. This position also allows for better digestion by facilitating the movement of food through the digestive system.

Avoid Tight-Fitting Clothing

Tight-fitting clothing can put pressure on the stomach, causing the LES to relax and allowing stomach acid to flow back up into the esophagus. To reduce symptoms of acid reflux, individuals should avoid wearing tight-fitting clothing, especially around the waist.

Quit Smoking

Smoking can contribute to acid reflux by increasing the production of stomach acid and causing the LES to relax. Quitting smoking can not only reduce symptoms of acid reflux but can also improve overall health.

Lifestyle modifications can play an important role in managing acid reflux disorder. By managing stress, exercising regularly, maintaining a healthy weight, elevating the head of the bed, sleeping on the left side, avoiding tight-fitting clothing, and quitting smoking, individuals can reduce symptoms of acid reflux and improve their overall digestive health. It is important to work with a healthcare professional to develop a personalized plan for managing acid reflux that takes into account individual triggers and symptoms. By making dietary and lifestyle changes, individuals can manage their acid reflux symptoms and improve their quality of life.

Chapter 7

Recipes for a Reflux-Friendly Diet: Delicious and Nutritious Meal Ideas for Breakfast, Lunch, Dinner, and Snacks that are Gentle on the Digestive System

In this chapter, we will provide some recipe ideas for a reflux-friendly diet that are both delicious and nutritious. These recipes are designed to be easy on the digestive system, with ingredients that are less likely to trigger acid reflux symptoms. Whether you're looking for ideas for breakfast, lunch, dinner, or snacks, these recipes are sure to satisfy your taste buds without causing discomfort.

Breakfast Ideas:

Oatmeal with Banana and Almond Milk
Ingredients:

1 cup rolled oats
1 cup almond milk

1 banana, sliced

1 tbsp honey (optional)

Instructions:

- In a small pot, combine the rolled oats and almond milk.
- Bring the mixture to a boil, then reduce the heat to low and simmer for 5-10 minutes or until the oatmeal is cooked to your liking.
- Top the oatmeal with sliced banana and drizzle with honey, if desired.

Greek Yogurt with Berries and Granola

Ingredients:

1 cup Greek yogurt

1/2 cup mixed berries (strawberries, blueberries, raspberries)

1/4 cup granola

Instructions:

In a bowl, add Greek yogurt.

Top with mixed berries and granola.

Lunch Ideas:

Grilled Chicken and Veggie Salad

Ingredients:

2 cups mixed greens

1 grilled chicken breast, sliced

1/2 cup cherry tomatoes, halved

1/2 cup sliced cucumber

1/4 cup crumbled feta cheese

2 tbsp balsamic vinaigrette

Instructions:

- In a large bowl, combine mixed greens, cherry tomatoes, sliced cucumber, and crumbled feta cheese.
- Top with sliced grilled chicken breast.
- Drizzle with balsamic vinaigrette.

- Roasted Vegetable and Quinoa Bowl

Ingredients:

1 cup cooked quinoa

1 cup roasted vegetables (zucchini, bell peppers, eggplant)

1/4 cup crumbled goat cheese

2 tbsp lemon vinaigrette

Instructions:

- In a bowl, add cooked quinoa.
- Top with roasted vegetables and crumbled goat cheese.
- Drizzle with lemon vinaigrette.

Dinner Ideas:

Baked Salmon with Roasted Asparagus

Ingredients:

4 oz salmon fillet

1/2 bunch of asparagus, trimmed

1 tbsp olive oil

1/2 tsp garlic powder

Salt and pepper to taste

Instructions:

- Preheat the oven to 400°F.
- On a baking sheet, add salmon fillet and asparagus.
- Drizzle with olive oil and season with garlic powder, salt, and pepper.

- Bake for 12-15 minutes, or until the salmon is cooked through and the asparagus is tender.

Turkey and Vegetable Stir-Fry

Ingredients:

4 oz ground turkey

1/2 cup sliced bell peppers

1/2 cup sliced zucchini

1/4 cup sliced onion

2 tbsp low-sodium soy sauce

1 tbsp sesame oil

1 tbsp cornstarch

Salt and pepper to taste

Instructions:

- In a large skillet, heat sesame oil over medium-high heat.
- Add ground turkey and cook until browned.
- Add bell peppers, zucchini, and onion to the skillet and stir-fry for 3-4 minutes, or until the vegetables are tender-crisp.
- In a small bowl, whisk together soy sauce and cornstarch.
- Pour the mixture over the stir-fry and stir until the sauce thickens.
- Season with salt and pepper to taste.

Snack Ideas:

Apple Slices with Almond Butter

Ingredients:

1 medium apple, sliced

2 tbsp almond butter

Instructions:

Spread almond butter on apple slices and enjoy.

Carrot Sticks with Hummus

Ingredients:

1 medium carrot, sliced into sticks

1/4 cup hummus

Instructions:

Dip carrot sticks into hummus and enjoy.

Conclusion

In this chapter, we provided some recipe ideas for a reflux-friendly diet that are both delicious and nutritious. By incorporating these meals into your diet, you can manage your acid reflux symptoms and improve your overall health. Remember to listen to your body and adjust your meals as needed to find what works best for you. With a little creativity and a willingness to try new foods, you can enjoy a reflux-friendly diet that doesn't sacrifice flavor or satisfaction.